Lifestyle
Change

Chris Dunn PhD
Acting Instructor
Department of Psychiatry and Behavioral Sciences,
University of Washington School of Medicine,
Seattle, WA,
USA.

Stephen Rollnick PhD
Professor of Healthcare Communication
Department of General Practice,
University of Wales College of Medicine,
Llaneydeyrn Health Centre,
Llaneydeyrn, Cardiff,
UK.

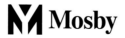

Dedications

Chris Dunn
For Ruth and Ellie, who are changing my behaviour more than any professional could.

Steve Rollnick
For Jacob, Stefan, Maya and Sheila.

MOSBY
An imprint of Elsevier Limited

The publisher's policy is to use paper manufactured from sustainable forests

© Elsevier Limited 2003. All rights reserved.

ISBN 0 7234 3318 6

Cataloguing in Publication Data
Catalogue records for this book are available from the US Library of Congress and the British Library.

Note
Medical knowledge is constantly changing. As new information becomes available, changes in treatment, procedures, equipment and the use of drugs become necessary. The editors, authors, contributors and the publishers have taken care to ensure that the information given in this text is accurate and up to date. However, readers are strongly advised to confirm that the information, especially with regard to drug usage, complies with the latest legislation and standards of practice.

Printed in China

Acknowledgements

We thank Pip Mason and Chris Butler for their support in the development of many of the strategies described in this book. Thanks to Peter Ways, MD, for his mentorship, careful manuscript reading, and wise advice.

Contents

Introduction

After you talk with a patient who is a smoker, are you usually satisfied or frustrated? For most practitioners, the answer depends upon the patient's response. If he seems ready and willing to change, then you may feel satisfied. But if he blames his addiction on the tobacco companies and refuses to budge, then you may feel frustrated. Or perhaps you avoided the topic altogether? Consider two examples with different outcomes from the same practitioner talking with the same patient.

You are seeing in clinic a 48 year-old man recovering from a recent heart attack and bypass surgery. He is still smoking after his surgery.

A good outcome:

Practitioner: Now that we have your medications straightened out, I'd like us to chat a bit about some lifestyle issues that can play a very important role in your recovery. Would that be all right?

Patient: *Sure. I'm already eating a little better than before and I've cut down on my smoking some.*

Practitioner: That's great news, and how is it going?

Patient: *Well, it's not earth shattering. I've only cut down from 25 cigarettes per day to around 18. But I was surprised at how easy it was to make that initial drop. I don't seem to miss those seven cigarettes at all yet.*

Practitioner: You must feel good about that, eh?

Patient: *It does feel good. My next goal is to get from 18 down to 12 over the next week by cutting away one more every day. I'm not using a patch or anything, and I'd actually like to get all the way to zero as soon as possible.*

Practitioner: Tremendous. At that rate, you'll be away from cigarettes soon.

Patient: *I don't know about that. I'm afraid it will get much harder as the number gets lower…I guess I'll just have to try it and see how things turn out.*

Practitioner: So you expect some tough times ahead, but you also seem very determined.

Patient: *Well, I know it's really very hard, especially to stay quit once you get there.*

Practitioner: Yes, and I believe you will make it. Remember, if you get stuck along the way, or decide you might like a little help, there are a few options you could choose from that work well for many people, such as a quit smoking class, or temporary medication.

Patient: *What's the class like?*

Practitioner: It's a group of people who get together once a week to help each other quit and stay quit. Some are in the process of setting quit dates and planning out their strategies, some are tapering like you are, and some are already abstinent. There happens to be a class this evening at the clinic if you are interested?

Patient: *Every week?*

Practitioner: Yes.

Patient: *I'm committed to something else tonight, but maybe I come next week? I should be down to only 12 cigarettes by then.*

Practitioner: That's great... I'll give you a brochure on the programme so you can learn more about it…Meanwhile, I'll do anything I can to help you as you go along. Please ask, okay?

Patient: *Sure, thanks.*

(Elapsed time: 2:30 minutes)

Comment

The practitioner asks permission to discuss lifestyle issues, and is quick to support the patient's initial efforts to quit. She assesses how confident the patient is, offers a menu of helpful options, and the patient chooses to try the quit smoking group. Medication options are left open. The next example involves the same practitioner (having a bad day!) and the same patient, but the practitioner talks differently and gets different results.

A not-so-good outcome:

Practitioner: Now that we have your medications straightened out, I'd like to go over a few lifestyle issues with you. They are as crucial to your recovery as the medications you are taking, perhaps more so.

Patient: *Sure. I'm already eating a bit better than before and I've cut down on my smoking some.*

Practitioner: I'm glad you mentioned that one, because smoking is the absolute worst thing you could do for your health now that you've had a heart attack. It's really quite serious.

Patient: *I'm down to 18 cigarettes a day…*

Practitioner: I'm afraid that's still way too much. The best way to deal with smoking is to take advantage of the fright this surgery has given you and quit right away, before you have time to change your mind. And the best way to quit and to stay quit is simply to set a quit date and stick to it.

Patient: *Well, I've been cutting down gradually because I don't like the sudden withdrawal caused by the cold turkey approach. I've tried that before and…*

Practitioner: Actually, the withdrawal lasts only a few days to a few weeks at its worst. Not much of a price to pay when you think about having another heart attack. As a matter of fact, there is a quit smoking class that meets here in the clinic this evening. What do you say?

Patient: *I've got something else to do tonight, and besides, I just need some time to think it over.*

Practitioner: Thinking will only prolong the inevitable. You're quite lucky that the class meets tonight. It's very successful, really. You show up, pick a quit date, and then stop. That's what you've got to do.

Patient: *That sounds like it might be helpful for some people, but I find I am quite uncomfortable in groups. You see I'm a bit of a loner and don't do too well in groups…*

(Elapsed time: 2:30 minutes)

Comment:

The practitioner ignores the patient's progress and issues a dire warning. She then prescribes the "best" way to quit, ignores the patient's concerns about withdrawal, suggests immediate action, and the patient digs in his heels.

How you talk with patients greatly affects the outcomes of these encounters. Try to exert control and your patient will seize it. Try to hurry things along and your patient will slow you down with "yes, buts". Choose for the patient which behaviour to work on, and the patient will change the topic or resist in some other way. In the end, the patient is the only one who can decide to change.

This book

This book is a Rapid Reference guide for understanding behaviour change counselling and for doing it even better than you do now. Our suggestions are derived from research and from our combined experience in teaching and performing behaviour change counselling with our own patients.

Much of the method in this book is adapted from Motivational Interviewing (MI), an evidence-based counselling style that helps people prepare for change.[1] This Rapid Reference book also draws heavily from Rollnick, Mason and Butler,[2] who have formulated a briefer version of MI for direct application in medical settings by practitioners who are not trained as counsellors. The method in this Rapid Reference book is called, "**behaviour change counselling**" (BCC). For a detailed discussion on the classification of different models of behaviour change methods, please see Rollnick, Allison, Ballasiotes et al.[3]

Part I offers our rationale for using behaviour change counselling in primary care settings, as well as evidence for its effectiveness. It also describes the basic differences between skilful and less skilful lifestyle counselling. Part II is about how to do it. It presents three main tasks constituting a successful behaviour change encounter, describing in detail how to do each one. These parts are as follows:

- **Raising the subject**
- **Exploring importance and raising confidence**
- **Discussing action options and closing**

Part III provides pragmatic tips for specific clinical situations encountered in daily primary care practice, including relapse and medication adherence discussions. Finally, the theory behind this book is summarised.

Part I

The rationale

It's a serious problem

Why bother?

The skilful consultation

It's a serious problem

Links between disease and unhealthy behaviour or inaction

The human brain has marvellously adapted for us to survive sudden danger. But why are so many people dying in slow motion due to excessive brain appetites for essential needs such as food, rest, or feeling good? Until neuroscience further solves this riddle, we are left to rely on behaviour change efforts. In simple terms, we must help our patients make decisions about stopping unhealthy behaviours and to starting healthy ones. Morbidity and mortality are inextricably linked to unhealthy patient behaviour or unhealthy inaction.

The three most prominent contributors to annual mortality in the United States in 1990: **smoking** (400,000 deaths), **unhealthy diet and activity patterns** (300,000), **excessive alcohol consumption** (100,000).[4]

- Over 120,000 deaths were caused by **smoking** in the UK in 1995; that is, one in five of all deaths.[5]
- **Smoking:** In 1998, 27% of adults aged 16 and over smoked cigarettes in England. Around 9% of children aged 11–15 smoke regularly.[5]
- **Coronary artery disease** accounts for one third of the 2 million American annual deaths.[6]
- **Smoking and high cholesterol** act synergistically to cause coronary artery disease.[7,8]
- **Diabetes:** 7 million Americans have diabetes, accounting for 11% of US health care expenditures.[9]
- **Obesity:** 55% of US adults are overweight, and two thirds of these overweight people have **diabetes**, heart disease, or **hypertension**.[10]
- **Inactivity:** One in 10 Americans die each year prematurely of medical problems that originate partly from physical inactivity.[11]
- Over one third of US adults with diabetes do not have adequate control over their blood pressure or lipid levels.[12]

- Glycaemic control: Less than half of patients with type 2 diabetes maintain HbA_{1c} < 7.0. Poor glycaemic control is related to inactivity, poor diet, and excessive alcohol consumption.[13]

- **Diabetes self-management:** In some populations, half of all patients have haemoglobin **HbA_{1c}** greater than 8%.[14]

- **Drugs use and HIV:** Among patients who are HIV positive, only 13% of active cocaine users maintained viral suppression, versus 46% of nonusers.[15]

- **Excessive drinking in England in 1998:** 20% of men and 8% of women had drunk more than 8 units of alcohol (6 units for women) on one or more days in the previous week. 27% of men and 12% of women had drunk more than 21 and 14 units a week respectively. 21% of pupils aged 11–15 had drunk in the previous week in 1999.[16]

- **Sun exposure:** Over 40% of adults in the UK who do not have naturally black or brown skin try to get tan and over 20% had been sunburned in the previous year.[17]

Box 1. The link between diseases and common "misbehaviours".

Links between improved behaviour and improved health

Happily, when people successfully maintain healthy behaviour changes, they greatly increase their chances of preventing, self-managing, and even reversing these prevalent medical problems. Patients may be encouraged by facts such those in Box 2.

Encouraging information to give to your patients

- **Diabetes:** Among patients with type 2 diabetes in the UK, for every 1% decrease in HbA1c, the risk of diabetes related death dropped 21% and the risk of micro vascular complications dropped 37%.[18]

- **Diabetes:** 12 exercise trials among patients with type 2 diabetes showed an overall decrease in HbA1c by 0.6%,[19] enough to reduce microvascular complications by 24%.[18]

Box 2. Encouraging information to give to your patients.

- **Diabetes prevention:** Among 3234 adults at high risk of developing type 2 diabetes (overweight, inactive and high fasting glucose), the incidence of diabetes onset over a 3-year period was 11.0% for a group receiving placebo, 7.8% for a group receiving metformin, and 4.8% for a group receiving a lifestyle intervention targeting **diet and exercise**.[20]
- After one year of abstinence, **smokers** reduce by 50% their chances of developing **coronary artery disease**.[9]
- After only a 30% reduction in alcohol consumption for one year, primary care patients who **drank excessively** reported improved physical and mental functioning, and reduced alcohol consequences.[21]
- **Blood pressure:** A low sodium diet can reduce systolic blood pressure by 7–11 mm Hg.[22]

Box 2. Continued.

But who should do behaviour change counselling?

We believe that all primary care health practitioners can be effective at behaviour change counselling. But for several reasons, many practitioners infrequently do this. One reason is *confidence*. They may not feel competent to influence behaviour, so they leave it up to the "behavioural specialists". *Aversion* is another reason. Many have tried it but stopped after suffering unpleasant encounters that damaged rapport with patients. A final barrier is limited *time* due to tight clinic scheduling.[23]

It is striking that reasons given by practitioners for not frequently performing behaviour change counselling are very similar to those given by patients for not increasing physical activity! For example:

- **Confidence:** I've tried to exercise regularly many times in the past, but it just never lasts.
- **Aversion:** When I try to walk more often, it only makes my feet ache more.
- **Time:** I'm a single mother. When I get home at night, I must cook and put the kids to bed. There just isn't time for exercise.

We have much in common with our patients, don't we?

Why bother?

It happens! Successful change occurs with or without help

Many patients successfully improve their lifestyles, and the health results range from subtle to spectacular. Surprisingly, more people successfully change their behaviour without professional help than with it.[24] A little help from us may be all they need to get going. And getting going—repeatedly—is what it takes to bring about lasting change. Even patients with very severe alcohol or drug problems who might need professional addiction treatment will benefit from a little help from their health care providers, because this effort can cause them to seek the help they need. Many practitioners have seen change emerge after years of sowing the seed.

Emphysemia: Mixtures of help

A 76 year-old man who had smoked for 60 years was diagnosed with emphysema and decided to quit smoking. He endured a tedious, self-paced reduction of daily cigarettes by recording them on his matchbook covers and plotting the daily tallies. Over 6 months, he dropped steadily by two cigarettes at a time from 35 per day to seven. At each step down point, he always waited for his confidence to rise before going lower. He then became depressed and was stuck at seven cigarettes per day. He reluctantly met with a psychiatrist, whom he described as "annoying". The psychiatrist failed to acknowledge this man's self-change attempt and insisted that his patient start with the *highest dose* patch, quit all seven cigarettes immediately, remain on the patch for 6 weeks, and start an antidepressant. ***Outcome:*** The man took the antidepressant, used only the *lowest dose* patch, and was abstinent within 2 weeks. He then threw away the rest of the patches, quit the antidepressant, and stop seeing his psychiatrist. He never smoked again. He said, *The drugs were very helpful; I'm not so sure about the psychiatrist.*

Box 3. Emphysemia: Mixtures of help.

> ### Diabetes and drinking
>
> A man with diabetes who has now abstained from drinking for 8 years attributes his success to the moment when his doctor briefly talked with him about his drinking 10 years ago. Looking back many years, this patient remembers only that the doctor was genuinely concerned and non-judgemental about his lack of readiness to change at the time. The patient saw this encounter as the turning point for him. It was 2 years after this encounter before he was sober.

Box 4. Diabetes and drinking.

Benefits of brief intervention

We use the term 'brief intervention' as a generic label. It refers to a variety of patient encounters requiring relatively little time and mostly providing brief advice rather then using counselling skills described in this book.

What is "behaviour change" and "behaviour change counselling" (BCC)?

We define behaviour change as any reduction in frequency or intensity of unhealthy behaviour or an increase in frequency or intensity of healthy behaviour. Practitioners should avoid rigid, all-or-nothing standards for deeming a behaviour change successful. Some change is always better than none, so take what you can get and be grateful!

To appreciate how widely the magnitude of behavioural change can vary, consider the following examples in Table 1. They differ in levels of commitment and levels of difficulty. Some of these examples of changes are "end points", others are intermediate goals or merely experiments to see what works.

In the primary care setting, we define "behaviour change counselling" (BCC) as any deliberate effort to use counselling skills to discuss behaviour (including medication use) with patients that encourages them to consider for themselves the why and the how of changing their behaviour. These encounters range in duration from a single encounter lasting 1 minute to a series of brief encounters spanning years. BCC can be performed by any practitioner of any discipline who cares enough and has the skill to do it. Behaviour change encounters are often called

Magnitude of behavioural changes	
Behaviour change	**Range of change magnitude**
Smoking	Quit entirely, reduce total daily cigarettes, cut out the "automatic" cigarettes that won't be missed, practice quitting by occasionally skipping the "most needed ones", e.g. delaying the first cigarette of the day.
Drinking	Quit entirely, reduce percentage of drinking days per month, reduce consumption per drinking day, practice abstinence by abstaining during selected occasions, alternate alcoholic with non-alcoholic beers.
Activity level	Exercise daily with strength, endurance, and flexibility training; exercising only 1 day per week, exercising on both weekend days only, adding stair climbing to your daily work routing, park far away and walk to the grocery store.
Eating better	Make a list of all binge foods and eliminate them, substitute low fat for high fat foods, make only one substitution at a time, eliminate eating within 2 hours of bedtime.
Safe sex	Always wear condoms during intercourse, reduce consumption of alcohol or drugs before sex, discuss your HIV status with sex partners.

Table 1. Magnitude of behavioural changes.

"opportunistic," because they occur in addition to the biomedical care for the patient's presenting concern. Practitioners often use an opportunistic intervention to link the behavioural change issue to the presenting concern (e.g. heavy drinking and stomach pain). These encounters may consist only of simple advice or education, although this book goes beyond that.

Effective drug therapies that help with behaviour change

The literature on the outcomes of brief intervention in primary care settings is growing rapidly. We offer the following conclusions about this literature, which are illustrated by the studies presented:

- Brief intervention accelerates natural change processes in people, thereby reducing the harm that would accrue during slower, unassisted change.

Outcomes of lifestyle counselling in primary care practice

- **Reducing alcohol consumption by brief counselling provided exclusively by physicians:** This study reviewed the 11 highest-quality randomized trials of brief counselling in medical facilities. Training for physicians lasted ≤ 1 hour. Counselling ranged from 2–30 minutes. Study follow-ups ranged from 4 months – 5 years, mostly one per year. **Results:** In the seven studies measuring drinks per week, patients receiving counselling reduced their weekly consumption by five;[25] seven;[26] seven;[27] 12;[28] and 20[29] more drinks than control group patients. Four of the eight studies measuring GGT levels showed greater declines in GGT for patients receiving counselling than for controls. Two of three studies measuring blood pressure reported significant decreases in systolic pressures for patients receiving counselling.[30]

- **Reducing alcohol consumption by brief counselling in medical settings:** In 11 of 12 randomized trials of brief counselling versus. no treatment across 14 nations improved referral or retention rates in specialist substance abuse treatment. Seven of eight trials of brief counselling without specialist treatment reduced consumption and/or alcohol-related problems. *"This places brief counselling among the most strongly supported intervention modalities for alcohol problems, and certainly as the most cost-effective, based on currently published clinical trials".*[31]

- **Smoking:** Reviewers of 188 randomized trials of smoking cessation interventions found that personal advice and encouragement to stop **given by physicians during a single routine consultation**, resulted in 2% (95% confidence limits, 1%, 3%; $p < .001$) of all patients quitting without relapse for up to 1 year. Advice and encouragement are more effective for patients who are pregnant (8% quit rate) or have ischaemic heart disease. *Behaviour modification techniques by behavioural specialists has equal effects but were several times more expensive.* Nicotine replacement therapy was effective in an estimated 13% of smokers who seek help to quit, and this effect is greatest for those most severely addicted. Arriving at abstinence by sudden cessation or by gradual reduction in smoking work equally well.[32]

- **Increasing physical activity:** 874 inactive men and women with no cardiovascular disease in US clinics were randomized to: **Recommended care:** 2–4 minutes physician advice +

written materials; **Telephone assistance:** Recommended care + lower intensity education and telephone counselling (3 hours total time over 2 years); **Counselling:** Recommended care plus higher intensity education and telephone counselling (9 hours total time over 2 years). **Results:** At the 2-year follow-up nearly all of the sample met physical activity guidelines (30 minutes moderate activity 5/week, or 30 minutes vigorous activity 3/week) compared to only 2% of sample at baseline. VO_2max: 5% increase at 24 months for women, no improvement for men. No advantage for more intensive counselling.[33]

- **Dietary intervention:** Meta-analysis of 17 randomized controlled trials of dietary behaviour interventions. **Result:** Compared to control group changes mean net changes over 9 to 18 months were: serum cholesterol, -0.22 (95% CI = -0.39, -0.05) mmol/L; urinary sodium, -45.0 (95% CI = -57.1, -32.8) mmol/24 hours; systolic blood pressure, -1.9 (95% CI = -3.0, 0.8) mm Hg; and diastolic blood pressure, -1.2 (95% CI = -2.6, 0.2) mm Hg. **Conclusions**. Individual dietary interventions in primary prevention can achieve modest improvements in diet and cardiovascular disease risk status that are maintained for 9 to 18 months.[34]

Box 5. Outcomes of lifestyle counselling in primary care practice.

- Skilful brief intervention consistently applied by primary care practitioners will produce behavioural change that translates into modest health gains that can collectively produce a large public health impact.
- People need continual reminders and support to sustain change, so never assume a patient's behavioural change effort is "over".

Medical technology continues to develop more effective drugs for helping patients to change unhealthy lifestyle behaviours. Several now exist that have helped many people, particularly for tobacco, heroin, and alcohol dependence. A few examples are listed in the appendix. An evaluation of the efficacy or safety of these agents is beyond the scope of this book.

The skilful consultation

This section presents the general ideas and methods of skilful behaviour change counselling. For more detailed "how to do it" information, see Part II.

A myth or more

Each of the following statements is clearly over-generalized and probably untrue. The implication is that *flexibility* in the consultation is a must.

- *There is a quick fix for behaviour change:* A review of the literature or an appraisal of healthcare delivery will readily reveal that no quick fix exists. Humility about what can be achieved is clearly warranted.
- *One approach will work for all:* Behaviour change consultations are a challenge precisely because patients are different, and have different needs.
- *Telling it to them straight is the only way:* Being clear in communication is a good thing. But "*telling them straight*" is much more than this. It's a behaviour change strategy based on direct persuasion. Patients often resist direct persuasion.
- *Time is all you need:* The issue of time can be oversimplified in defence of poor practice.

Practitioner thoughts: I don't have the time to spend 20 minutes on lifestyle change with my patients. My job is to tell them what I think, give them some advice, and move on.

One patient's experience of the briefest of interventions: *When I was a young man, I smoked and had bronchitis. I went to the doctor for an X-ray and the results were negative. I told the doctor I smoked, and he said that maybe that prevented my bronchitis from clearing. As he was leaving the room, I was putting on my shirt. He paused and with a tone of genuine curiosity, he said, "Hmm. You look too healthy to be a smoker". He wasn't* *judging me, nor lecturing. It hit me right between the eyes. From that moment forward, I knew I wasn't living in accordance with my values. That's all. I'll never forget it. I haven't smoked in 22 years.*

(Elapsed time of intervention: 3 seconds)

There will be occasions when time is tight, and other times when it is less so. There will be patients whom you decide to spend a little more time with, and those with whom you decide not to do this. There is no single solution for all patients. Lots of time can be *wasted* in delivering advice to the unreceptive patient. Listening can save time.

Say less, achieve more

Doing less yourself is probably more important than anything else. It means that the patient will be doing more. A patient who is active in the consultation will be more likely to change. Achieving this usually means listening and understanding rather than telling or persuading.

The clumsy consultation

A clumsy consultation can have serious consequences, as illustrated in the next two examples of consent for surgery. In primary care, the outcomes of skilful and less skilful encounters may be less immediate and dramatic, but equally important in the long run.

Please sign this form or else

One of our own students was on a very busy ward round with a group of nine practitioners. They stopped at the bedside of a middle-aged woman with diabetes who had been warned that her leg might need to be amputated. Still clearly distressed, she couldn't agree to the strong advice given to her to sign the consent form. The doctor said, *I am afraid to say that if you don't sign the form the implications could be serious. You might even die.* Her response was, *But I just can't live with one leg, I can't do it.* The group moved on, and the student learned a few days later that she had not signed the form and had died.

Box 6. Consequences of a clumsy consultation.

A skilful consultation, different outcome

A team of rehabilitation specialists visited a patient with lower leg gangrene to convince him to consent to an immediate below the knee amputation. The patient dug in his heels and refused, despite the surgeon's best attempt at compassionate persuasion. The man became more and more agitated, so the team left. An hour later, one team member visited the patient. She asked him to tell her his view of the pros and cons of the surgery. She simply listened to both sides of his view and summarized what she had heard. His belief was that a below the knee prosthesis would cause a bad limp. Once the patient had finished speaking (3 minutes), the physician asked permission to give him some information. It was that such a prosthesis enables a near-perfect stride pattern, that people have run marathons on these devices. She left the room and encouraged the patient to take more time to think about it. The patient buzzed the front desk within an hour and consented to the procedure.

Box 7. A skilful consultation.

The basic ideas behind a skilful consultation

Reactance

According to reactance theory, people resist suggestions not because of the rational content of your suggestion, but because their freedom to make decisions is being taken away.[35] No one likes that, so resistance erupts.

Time for your bath, Ellie (2 years old)

Mother: *Time for your bath, Ellie* (with jubilance)

Child: No... (calmly, matter-of-factly)

Mother: (enthusiastically) *Look! I'm putting Pixie and Mary (waterproof dolls) in first!*

Child: No, no.(more firmly)

Mother: *But Pixie and Mary can't take a bath all by themselves; they need your help, sweetie!* (a desperation attempt at rational persuasion)

Child: No, no, NO! (firing the warning shot across the bow)

Mother: (leaving Ellie no choice) *Honey,* (takes Ellie's hand) *come with me, please. You know how much fun baths are...*

Ellie: (screaming): NO!!!!!!!!!

(Elapsed time to meltdown: 24 seconds)

Avoiding resistance initially takes longer than arousing resistance; but avoiding resistance can save time in the long run. Avoid arousing reactance.

Box 8. Arousing resistance.

Readiness, importance and confidence

A few concepts specific to the subject of behaviour change are worth considering the next time a patient seems reluctant to change. Ambivalence—feeling two ways about change—is very common. Patients vary in their readiness to change, and it is useful to think of readiness on a continuum. Many patients are around the midpoint of this continuum–ambivalent! [36] If you jump ahead of their readiness by talking to them as if they should be more ready and give them advice to change, they will resist. The art of the behaviour change consultation is to understand how ready a patient is, and start there. If a patient does not get to the point of decision-making about change, it does not mean that the consultation has failed. Just talking through the pros and cons can be very useful.

Two further concepts can be useful for understanding why a patient is perhaps not so ready to change. This might be because change is not particularly important, or it might have to do with confidence. Each of these can be placed on a continuum, and Figure 1 illustrates their relationship to readiness. Put simply, high importance and high confidence will probably mean that the patient is nearly ready to change. [2]

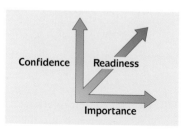

Figure 1. Confidence and importance — the relationship with readiness.

Aids to flexible behaviour change counselling

Using open questions

Some experienced practitioners tell us that, as the years go by, their open questions get shorter and shorter. Why? How? What? are probably the most common words used in open questions, which ensure that the patient is unlikely to reply with a simple yes or no answer: What makes you say you want to eat better? How might you accomplish this?

Long and short summaries

Long summaries, where you simply gather together your understanding of the patient's situation and experience, are used at key junctures in the consultation. They allow you to steer the conversation to the tasks of behaviour change.[2] The patient will feel understood and therefore be more agreeable about a change in topic. Example of a long summary: So on one hand, you realize you're putting yourself in danger by not using condoms, but on the other hand, you're not sure it's worth going to the trouble. Instead, you're more inclined to rely on a spermicide. (Summary allows changing directions): Would it be all right if I gave you a bit of information about spermicide and viruses? For more examples of long summaries, see pages 41 & 50.

Short summaries are a de-jargonized variant of empathic listening. They are more difficult to use skilfully, and involve briefly summarising your understanding of what the patient is saying and experiencing continually during the encounter. Summaries have the effect of encouraging the patient to amplify their account, and are particularly useful when you have asked an open question and wish the patient to continue with the answer.[2] Examples of short summaries: You're not too happy about hearing your blood sugar is high…Seems like you've been trying hard…

Further reading on this topic can be found in Miller & Rollnick[1] and Rollnick, Mason, & Butler.[2]

Elicit-Provide-Elicit (E-P-E): Exchanging information

As our patient walks out, we all seriously wonder how much

information has been absorbed. One additional guideline that might help is the *Elicit-Provide-Elicit* framework.[2] Sometimes it takes a little more time to use it. Sometimes one can waste less time because by not giving information that the patient either does not want or already knows.

- **E**licit what the patient wants to know and does know.
- **P**rovide information.
- **E**licit the patient's reactions.

For examples of this method, see pages 39 & 46–47.

Handling resistance and avoiding debate

Resistance is patient behaviour in the consultation that indicates unwillingness to go along with your suggestions. It can take many forms: denial, passivity, saying "Yes, but…", or even appearing to agree with what you say. How then can you detect it? Trust your judgement. You can use the "gut meter": the less good you feel about what a patient says, the more likely that remark is a resistant one. Others call this sense the "third eye", because as you talk, your third eye watches how things are going and adjusts, if resistance arises.

In general, *the better the rapport you have, the less the likelihood of resistance emerging.*

Resistance is often a signal for you to change direction, in order to improve rapport. Consider any of the following strategies:

- Summarize what the patient has said and even how you think they might be feeling.
- Give the patient some freedom to decide what to talk about or where to go next.
- Check with the patient to see if you have offended him, and remind him that you are not going to push him toward changes he doesn't want to make.
- Try a simple, non-dramatic apology: *Sorry, I didn't mean to push on you, it truly is up to you to decide if and when to take action.*

Advice giving

A tired, routine line of patter is quite different from a carefully timed, well-delivered piece of advice. Both options require the

Raising the subject and getting going

Getting going can be the hardest task

Some providers don't raise the subject of behaviour change for good reasons. Many avoid the subject to be polite or to respect their patients' privacy. They may rightly judge that the time is not right. Other priorities prevail.

Asthma medication non-adherence

- *I'm quite sure this patient is not regularly using his inhaler to prevent asthma attacks. I bet if I raise the subject he will just tell me what I want to hear.*
- *All I can do is offer my professional advice, and if he chooses not to take his medication, that's his business, that's as far as I go…*
- *Besides, I don't want to put him off by foisting this issue upon him…*

Box 10. Raising the subject.

How you approach patients will strongly influence how frankly they explore the topics of lifestyle change with you. *Starting slowly saves time later on, because it minimises resistance.* The first few words you exchange shape the trajectory of the ensuing discussion. The patient might relax, let you in on this private part of his life and seriously explore change. Or he might clam up, resist, and resent the intrusion.

There are many ways to get over a few early hurdles. If you put a little time aside and follow the guidelines below, you might sort out this issue once and for all.

There are no rigid formulae for doing this. But we suggest you consider three things which we have found practitioners can easily accomplish in a sentence or two:

- Make sure it is it okay to discuss this topic with the patient.
- Be explicit that this will be a very brief discussion.

- Does the patient understand you will not insist on immediate action?

  Example: I would like to take just a few minutes to get a better idea of how you are using your inhaler. Don't worry, I won't be lecturing you, okay?

Asking to dance—to avoid wrestling

Raising the subject skilfully is a social convention, like asking permission to dance. Rather than abruptly grabbing her hand and pulling her onto the dance floor, it is best to first ask her if she would like to dance. This ensures that you will be dancing and not wrestling. Good BCC feels more like dancing than wrestling (Jeff Allison, personal communication).

Box 11. Skilfully raising the subject.

Strategy: Using a menu of topics to raise the subject

Unhealthy lifestyle behaviours usually occur in clusters. At any particular moment, people are more ready and willing to change some behaviours than others. Consider the diabetic patient who is inactive, smokes and has a risky diet. You might be tempted to pick the topic by yourself: *"Let's have a look at your smoking, because that is by far the most dangerous thing you could be doing.* But this may bog down quickly: "*Actually, I couldn't possibly quit smoking right now. There are just too many pressures for me to deal with these days"* (low importance, low confidence).

Option 1: Offer a menu of topics to choose from… "I have in mind a few things that can affect how good you feel, among them smoking, exercising, and drinking alcohol. Which of these might be important for you to discuss? Or is there something else on your mind that seems more important?"

Option 2: Show patients the diagram[38] in Figure 2. Each circle symbolizes a lifestyle behaviour and you simply ask your patient if he is interested in discussing any of these topics. A few circles on the chart are also left empty, so the patient can raise his own concerns as well. Offering a menu of topics makes the patient responsible to decide what to discuss. If you have an urgent topic that in your view cannot be skipped, then get agreement to discuss both.

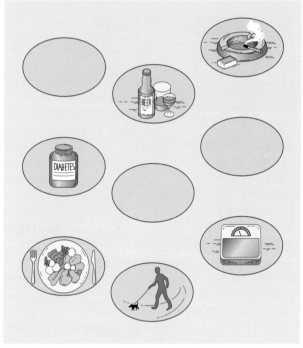

Figure 2. Stott's diagram.

Tips for raising the subject

We illustrate these tips using examples of patients whom you suspect are drinking too much alcohol but they apply to all behaviours. Patients with the most severe alcohol problems are easiest to notice. You see them, may sense that they are overwhelmed by alcohol dependence, even smell them. With others, your concern is milder. Yet how do you raise the subject with someone who does not want to talk about it, or so you believe?

If the patient alludes to the topic: This allows you to direct the discussion back to alcohol when you have a chance… *"A moment ago, you mentioned that you usually have a few glasses of wine with dinner, and one before bed. Is it okay if we explore the topic of drinking a little? I won't try to push you into making any changes you're not okay with. What do you say?"*

If the patient's presenting concern (e.g. insomnia) is linked to excessive drinking: Ask your patient what she knows about this link and then add information to make that link explicit. *"While we're on the topic of waking early and not dropping off to sleep again, I'd like you to tell me what you already know about how alcohol can affect sleep. Is that okay?"*

If your patient mentions stress: Assess whether your patient sees alcohol as a means of coping with stress. If so, you can explore other ways to cope without drinking …*You mentioned you are under a huge amount of stress these days. What have you found so far that is helpful for handling this pressure?*

Getting out of a common pothole: Hitting early resistance

If you probe an inflamed appendix too aggressively, this can cause subsequent guarding during the examination. Raising the topic of behaviour change too abruptly can have the same effect. It is common to encounter early defensiveness but this is usually easy to repair to get back on track. Consider these two examples.

HIV: raising the subject of safe sex

A 29 year-old man with HIV who has sex with men:

Pr: **Now that we have your medications straightened out, is it okay with you if we discuss an important lifestyle issue concerning sex?**

Pa: What do you mean?

Box 12. Discussing HIV.

Exploring importance and raising confidence

A simple strategy

As presented in detail elsewhere,[2] this simple strategy guides many clinicians carrying out BCC. You assess importance and confidence. It is only a guide, not a lockstep prescription for what to do. In real life discussions, importance and confidence are sometimes woven together. Or you may prefer using words such as "commitment", "intention", "optimism", or "hope". The point is that merely exploring importance and confidence can increase readiness and that's what a successful brief intervention does.

Three questions for exploring importance and confidence

The same three questions can assess both importance and confidence.[2] The generic versions of these questions appear just below, followed by specific clinical examples of their use. Notice the rich information they yield.

Exploring importance

- Question 1: *I'd like to understand how important it is to you personally to (**make the change under discussion**). If 0 is not important and 10 is very important, what number would you give yourself?*
- Question 2: *Why did you give it a (**whatever number the patient gave it**) and not a (**lower number than the patient gave**)?*
- Question 3: *What would it take for you to give it a (**higher number than the patient gave**)?*

Exploring confidence

- Question 1: *I'd like to understand how confident you are that if you were to decide to (**make the change under*** *discussion), that you would be successful. If 0 is not at all confident and 10 is very confident, what number would you give yourself?*

- Question 2: *Why did you give it a (**whatever number the patient gave it**) and not a (**lower number than the patient gave**)?*
- Question 3: *What would it take for you to give it a (**higher number than the patient gave it**)?*

Exploring importance

Pr: I'd like to understand how important is it to you personally to make a change in your smoking. If 0 was not important and 10 was very important, what number would you give yourself?

Pa: I'd say it is about a 8.

Pr: And why did you give it an 8 and not a 3?

Pa: Because I know I might get cancer and I'd miss lots of time with my grandchildren.

Pr: So being around to watch them grow up is crucial to you.

Pa: Yes, very much so.

Pr: And what would it take for you to give quitting say, a 9 or 10 in importance?

Pa: I'd have to be sure that I could at least succeed in quitting for the first few day, and stay sane....

Box 14. Exploring importance.

Tips for raising importance and confidence

Exchanging information to raise importance

Information is handy for raising the importance of change by adding to patients' concerns about the status quo (e.g. negative consequences). We don't provide any extra examples here, because most practitioners have plenty of bad news to give

Exploring the pros and cons of going without condoms (status quo)

A man who is HIV positive and has multiple sex partners mentioned earlier that he seldom uses condoms. You choose to explore the status quo rather than change:

Pr: I'd like to understand more about how you feel about using condoms or not using them. Would that be all right?

Pa: Sure, I know this is very important to doctors...

Pr: Right. I do think it's important. But what matters more is how you feel about it. First of all, what are the things that you like about not wearing a condom?

Pa: Well, most men know that sex is more pleasurable without a condom. And, I don't have to bother with the awkwardness of discussing it with a new partner.

Pr: I see. It feels better physically and things go more smoothly if you don't bother to wear one. (A short summary.) Other things you like about not using one?

Pa: That's mostly it, I guess.

Pr: And what about the other side of the picture for you. What do you not like about the idea of going without condoms?

Pa: Well, I do think it's my partner's responsibility to ask if he is concerned, really. But I guess it would be partly my fault if I were to infect someone else...

Pr: So on one hand, it's more pleasurable and comfortable not to bother, but on the other hand, you wouldn't want anyone else to contract HIV from you. Is that about right? (A nice summary of both pros and cons.)

Box 17. Exploring the pros and cons – an example.

Exploring the pros and the cons

Exploring the pros and cons of the status quo (the problem behaviour) is another way to understand your patient's views on importance and confidence. This activity is engrossing, and we find that patients work hard to articulate both sides of their ambivalence. Your task is to structure this brief exploration by doing the following:

- Elicit the pros.
- Elicit the cons.
- Summarize.

The patient's task is to help you understand how she sees this conflict. This will likely differ from your views.

Note: You can either ask about the pros and cons of the status quo or the pros and cons of changing. There is no formula for which approach to use. Either approach will elicit the patient's view. We suggest that if you sense reluctance to change, then discuss the status quo; if you sense a desire to change, then discuss change. See the example in Box 17, on page 40

Examples of summaries of ambivalent patients' views

The diabetic patient hesitant to start taking insulin: *Let me see if I understand what you have said. On one hand, you aren't too sure you really need insulin, because you've got along fine without it for many years, until just recently when your feet became numb. On the other hand, you are quite concerned that something else might happen if you don't get your sugar under control again. Have I missed anything?*

The obese, inactive patient: *Overall, you're really not interested just now in beginning regular exercise. You're working hard on your diet, you only recently quit smoking, and you are taking care of two extra children for the summer months, which steals most of your free time. Is that about it?*

The hesitant, heavy drinker: *So you seriously considering quitting drinking, but you still have your doubts that you even need to do this, because you're convinced you're not an alcoholic.*

Box 18. Examples of summaries.

Getting out of common potholes

Cheerleading: the HbA$_{1c}$ cheer
Cheerleading results when the good-hearted practitioner gets "finish line fever". This can lead to "deciding for her" that change is important and attainable rather than letting her arrive at these decisions for herself. Supportive enjoyment is good, but one can get carried away

Stuck in an awkward moment From time to time we all get stuck in awkward moments when discussing lifestyle change. Maybe the patient suddenly becomes defensive and you can't figure out why. He might change the topic abruptly in an obvious effort to stop the discussion. Or you might notice that both of you are suddenly tense and quiet. When in doubt, *make the obvious explicit.*

Discussing action options and closing

But I shouldn't discuss action with less ready patients, true?

It is true that discussing action prematurely can result in your patient becoming resistant and dragging behind. But **how** you discuss action will determine how your patient responds. With less ready patients, this can be done as a "hypothetical look over the fence".[2] In other words, If you were to decide one day to change, how do you think you might go about it?

Discussing action with a patient who is not quite ready can clarify his goals. Hypothetical talk helps him to imagine how a change would specifically happen if and when he were to take action. Imagining a tangible goal and tangible plan can raise confidence because the task then seems more achievable. As mentioned previously, if your "gut meter" tells you things are not going well, you are probably too far ahead of your patient's readiness.

Asking the key question

You have explored your patient's view of importance and confidence, and summarized it accurately. You are now at a turning point: either close on good terms (see the end of this section), or move ahead to discussing a plan. To determine which it will be, ask the key question along the lines of, **Where does all this leave you now?**[1]

Responses that indicate it's time to move further into discussing action are:

- I'm determined to make a change. (*strong commitment*)
- Well, I don't know. It's high time I did something about this, I'm just not sure what. (*less commitment, but open to exploration*)

- I'm not planning on having a drink any time soon, now that I have this stomach problem. *(less strong commitment but still worth pursuing)*

Responses that indicate it's time to close on good terms are:

- I don't know. I guess I just have to do some serious thinking before I say I'm going to make any changes.
- Thanks for your concern, but I'm not ready to take the plunge just yet.
- I just don't think it's a problem.

Discussing a plan

This involves brainstorming, meaning that all ideas are welcomed, no matter how unrealistic. The E-P-E method for exchanging information (page 27) is very helpful for discussing a plan. First *elicit* (E) what the patient thinks he should do, then *provide* (P) your own opinion, then *elicit* (E) his personal response to it. As discussed later in Part II, if your patient has made a previous change effort(s) and relapsed, this plan must be a new-and-improved-one. Once people believe that they have a solid plan, they feel more confident.

Clarify goals: First, help your patient to choose a behavioural goal. To do this, simply ask what her specific goals are. Does she want to reduce fats and sweets in her diet, or only sweets?

Discussing a plan for change using E-P-E

A middle-aged man with diabetes, with poorly controlled sugars and elevated HbA1c. (The practitioner has already elicited and summarised the patient's views on losing weight):

Pr: (the key question): **So where does all this leave you now?**

Pa: Well, I've certainly got to lose some weight.

Pr: (clarifying goals): **Great. What do you think would be a reasonable amount to lose in, say, two months?**

Pa: Thirty pounds, at least.

Pr: (setting a reasonable goal): That's quite a lot, actually. You might choose a lower goal for the short run, such as 5 or 10 pounds in 2 months. You can always raise your goal in 2 months.

Pa: Right. Okay, 10 pounds seems reasonable.

Pr: (Elicit): What are your ideas about how you might do this?

Pa: I certainly need to remind myself how important it is to lose weight. And no fat or sweets. No eating just before bedtime, either. (unrealistic expectation).

Pr: (Provide): Those are excellent ideas. And exerting your will is certainly important. Do you mind if I toss out a few other things that work well for my patients?

Pa: Sure.

Pr: To get a solid start, people do well if they can think of one or two specific foods which they replace with something healthier? (Elicit): What do you think of that approach?

Pa: Yes...iced cream and French fries. I know those are two major downfalls.

Pr: (Elicit): Great. So let's think of a few healthy things to substitute, ones that really are satisfying...

Box 21. Discussing a plan for change.

If she chooses an extremely difficult goal, you can help her to adjust it until it is attainable and specific.

Note: When clarifying goals, help your patient to set *realistic, obtainable* ones. Patients often have unrealistic expectations of what can be achieved and how easy it will be to achieve them. See later for a discussion of self-efficacy versus overconfidence.

Reach an agreement, no matter what

So that you both feel good about the session and will be more likely to repeat it in the future, always "reach an agreement". This agreement may not include the patient's commitment to begin immediate action, because so many patients are not that ready. Some important intermediate outcomes are:

- Agreeing to watch the behaviour in question rather than change it immediately.
- Agreeing to discuss the topic with a health counsellor or other professional.
- Agreeing to think about it.
- Agreeing to amicably disagree with each other about the need for change.
- Agreeing to write a list of the pros and cons of changing.

Is merely agreeing to think about change a successful outcome? If that's all you can get, and if you both feel good about how the consult went, then yes.

Mental rehearsal improves follow-through

For more ready patients who have genuine intentions to take action, a simple method has been shown to work. To do this, help your patient to form a simple plan: *"Whenever situation X arises, I will take my medicine."* Situation X is the anticipated trigger that already occurs automatically in that patient's life, such as going outside for the morning paper. Linking a new behaviour to a daily, automatic behaviour automatically implements the intention. Once the decision to do the new behaviour is "put on autopilot", action is easier.[39] This strategy has been found to numerous lifestyle behaviours, among them vitamin intake[40] attendance at cervical cancer screening[41] and regular exercise.[39]

Closing on good terms

A successful consult ends on good terms and when the time is right. A skilful closing can determine how future discussions with this patient will go. Patients vividly remember both pleasant and unpleasant encounters vividly. Closing on good terms gives you a chance to offer final praise and encouragement. It's up to you to find something they did well during the consult and praise them for doing it. The following acronym may help to form a good summary:

    S: Summarize your patient's views on importance and confidence.

A mental rehersal for exercising:

An elderly woman with elevated blood pressure and very mild depression has the intention to begin exercising regularly.

Pr: It can help to mentally rehearse your plan to exercise. Okay?

Pa: Sure.

Pr: You said you have thought of taking a daily walk with your neighbour.

Pa: (identifying the automatic behaviour already established): Right. She and I have been talking about that. Every morning, I go out to get the paper and then knock on her door. She always has some coffee on and we sit in her kitchen and have a cup together.

Pr: Sounds like you don't ever forget to do that!

Pa: No, we kid ourselves about having such great discipline that we never miss our morning cup!

Pr: How about linking to this morning ritual to a morning walk?

Pa: What do you mean?

Pr: (linking to an automatic behaviour): If you both made a solid pact, you could take a lap around the block together while the coffee is brewing. Perhaps even a solemn pledge: no short walk, no coffee?

Pa: (laughing) Right, we could nudge each other that way.

Box 22. Mental rehearsal.

E: Earnestly praise your patient for work done during the encounter.

W: What agreement was reached is underlined.

Tips for closing on good terms

- Closing can happen at any time during the consult.
- It's not how many things you did during the consult that matters.
- What matters is that you both enjoyed a brief dance and would do it again.

A good summary and closing

A woman with asthma who frequents the emergency room several times per year is not yet ready to commit to using her inhaler regularly:

Pr: (Summary of patient's views on importance and confidence): You'd very much like to avoid the emergency room in the future, and you understand how using your inhaler can help. On the other hand, you're not sure you want to go to the trouble of making this a habit, even though you feel confident that you could actually remember to do it if you decided to. You're not alone in feeling this way. Most people need to think and talk about it more before they decide.

Pa: I know I should use it more often, but I just can't make myself focus on that right now, the rest of my life is in such chaos at the moment...

Pr: (Earnest praise): Great. Let's stop here for now, and thanks for having that brief chat with me. You're really taking this seriously, I can tell. The important thing is you haven't shut your mind to the possibility.

Pr: (What was agreed to): You said you're going to start keeping track of how often you do use it, and think about some more convenient ways to use it more often. That's a great start. Is it okay if we briefly touch on this next visit to see how it's going?

Pa: Okay, thanks

Box 23. A useful summary and closing statement.

- Acknowledge uncertainty and reassure patients that it is normal.
- Be optimistic that change is possible.
- Reassure patients that ambivalence is normal.
- Praise patients for not being overly confident.
- Ask to dance again in the future.

■ Part III ■

Pragmatics and theory

Tips for specific behaviours
and situations

Relapse and recovering
commitment to change

Medication adherence

The world of theory
and evidence

I can stop anytime I want

A 42 year-old man who is a carpenter presents with belly pain, with gradual onset over the past 3 months. He smokes, has a distended gut, and possibly extended liver margins on examination. You suspect that drinking might contribute to the problem:

Pr: (raising the topic skilfully): It would help me to better understand your lifestyle if you could tell me a bit about your drinking...

Pa: I don't drink that often; I go for days without drinking at all. I just like to have a few beers now and then. I don't have a problem with it. I never get drunk or anything like that. And I can stop any time I want. (alert: immediate resistance)

Pr: (roll with resistance by praising the good in his message): Good. It sounds like you pay careful attention to your drinking and you know it can be serious for some people.

Pa: Right. I've got some friends who are pretty bad off and I don't intend ever to get that way. My dad was like that; he died of liver failure...

Pr: You can clearly see that it hurt him, eh?

Pa: Right. He drank every day for years. Like right now, since my belly began to hurt worse, I haven't had a drink in 3 or 4 days. Nothing. (You now sense that he drinks quite heavily at times. Let go of that, it will only damage rapport.)

Pr: I wonder if we might explore this together by running a few tests that will help us sort out your belly pain.

Pa: Like what?

Pr: I'd like to run some blood tests and discuss the results with you next week. We'll check your liver functions, find out your cholesterol levels, things like that. It will help me to track down your belly pain. And, it's an opportunity to make sure you're not running into any of the troubles your father might have had. What do you say? (Findings such as elevated GGT or MCV might be future information to raise importance.)

Pa: Sure, anything to get rid of this pain.

Pr: Good then. I'll see you next week and we can go over the results...

Box 24. Difficult situations.

Tips for specific clinical situations

1. *I can stop any time I want; therefore, I do not have a drinking problem:* Have you heard this often? You inquire politely about his drinking and he immediately presents his well-polished lines to convince you that he's a normal drinker.

Many people who drink excessively experience lengthy periods of sobriety or moderation, without much effort. These intervals are followed by periods of heavier consumption, forming what can be a life-long cycle of ebb and flow. These people seldom consider themselves to "have a drinking problem". Maybe they started to feel some loss of control, but by returning to moderation or abstinence their sense of control was renewed. They may think of someone "with a drinking problem" as an addicted person only to be the heavy, daily drinker with strong withdrawal symptoms. In the United States at least, "a drinking problem" is a euphemism for near total loss of control.

2. The question–answer pothole: This trap is a pattern of talking that quickly makes the practitioner work harder than the patient. It shifts the responsibility for change from patient to practitioner. This trap is easy to fall into and can result from leading the dance with too heavy a hand…

3. Mismatching agendas pothole: Presenting patients with a menu of behavioural topics can identify the behaviour the patient is most ready to discuss. But sometimes this is overlooked and must be repaired…

4. *Why don't you…, Yes, but…* **pothole:** You delicately suggest that the patient might need to reduce weight. For good reason. In return, you receive the *"Yes, but…"* response. The patient tells you why that is not a good idea, or why it will never work.

Getting out: *Emphasize autonomy: I know you've worked hard at this before and had some discouraging moments. And*

The question–answer pothole

A 39 year-old female smoker with HTN who presents with a bad cold and HTN.

Pr: **How much are you smoking?**

Pa: Hardly at all, with this cold.

Pr: **Have you ever quit?**

Pa: Once

Pr: **For how long?**

Pa: A few weeks.

Pr: **Did you use the patch?**

Pa: No.

Pr: **And what about trying bupropion, have you ever tried that?**

Pa: No, I don't believe in taking drugs unnecessarily...

(the practitioner working too hard and it takes too long to understand her view on smoking this way)

Getting out: *Relinquish the lead*. If you catch yourself asking rapid-fire questions, ***shift from asking to summarizing***. The patient will then begin to explore the topic with you, rather than merely fend off your questions.

Pr: **(summary): Okay. So when you have a cold you smoke less, and you have managed to quit once for a few weeks without the help of the patch.**

Pa: Yeah. I know I need to quit someday but it's hard to try again after I failed that one time.

Pa: That surely can be discouraging. (it may now be possible to ask the "key question" and discuss action options.

Box 25. The question and answer trap.

I won't blame you if you decide that it's not worth a go. It's completely up to you; but I'll help in any way possible. What do you think?

5. Providing single, simple solutions pothole: Many practitioners fall into the habit of providing single, simple solutions. A patient seems quite ready to consider a change. So

Mismatching agendas pothole: diabetes, smoking, and diet

This patient was recently diagnosed with type 2 diabetes. The practitioner prematurely focuses on smoking, hits resistance, and then repairs nicely.

Pr: Now that we have adjusted your medications, I would like to talk about some of the things in your lifestyle that can help greatly to manage your diabetes. And the first thing that comes to mind is smoking.

Pa: I don't smoke nearly as much as in the past.

Pr: How much are you smoking now? (focusing on quantity-frequency)

Pa: About half a pack a day, maybe a little more…

Pr: I see. Well, as you know, diabetes is a disease of the blood vessels, and even smoking half a pack a day is one of the most dangerous things you could be doing to your health.

(pursuing the topic without patient's agreement and announcing for the patient how important she should consider quitting smoking to be.)

Pa: Uh huh. I know. But there are so many things to deal with right now, my diet, exercising more, taking all those medicines… I'm just not ready to rush into quitting smoking right now.

Getting out:

Pr: (repairing by renegotiating the topic): Mmm. I'm sorry to be pushing a bit hard just then. Perhaps we could leave the smoking for now and get back to it at some future date? (Summarising what the patient said): You mentioned you are aware of several things at the moment that will help you manage your diabetes. Which of these seems most important to you currently?

Pa: I've been trying to think of low-fat foods to substitute for some of the high-fat things I have eaten in the past.

Pr: That's really great. What ideas have you come up with so far?…

Box 26. Dealing with mismatching agendas.

you make a single, constructive suggestion about how they might go about this. This is often phrased in a closed question: *Have you ever thought of…* The response you get is resistance. *That simply doesn't work for me…*

Getting out: *Provide multiple solutions and encourage choice:* The way out of this is fairly straightforward; it simply involves mentioning more than one solution, and encouraging the patient to select one that seems most suitable: *Everyone is different. Some people do X, some do Y or Z. What about you, what do you think makes the most sense?*

Relapse and recovering commitment to change

Healthy thoughts to think about relapses

Often, we practitioners are the first to "relapse" within the change partnership. That is, after helping patients to act, we presume that the problem is gone. We withdraw support by not helping patients to solidify their commitment to maintain change. Helping patients maintain change involves repeatedly raising the topic and praising our patients for the gains they have made.

> Sarah M, a patient with obesity and hypertension, was proud of her 7 kilogram weight loss and had enjoyed two doctor visits during which her blood pressure was normal. But now, 7 months later, her excess weight has returned and her blood pressure is elevated again. It is as if she had never changed her behaviour at all. She feels that she has failed, and she is ready to conclude that her situation is hopeless.

Box 27. A problem of relapse.

Once they have returned to their old ways, patients usually despair. As practitioners, we tend to despair also. Our worst doubts about our patient are now confirmed: she never wanted to change badly enough; or worse, she'll never succeed because she lacks what it takes.

To help such an individual prepare for another change effort, we must first regain our own optimism. To do this, there is no need to become polyannish. Most patients who eventually enjoy lasting change–without relapses—attain this after weathering several relapses. In a survey of former problem drinkers who now have an average of 13 years of continuous sobriety, one in three made at least *three serious attempts* to stop before they were successful; one in five had to try five or more times.[43]

The natural history of relapses: they come and go, then finally, go

Often but not always, relapse is a natural part of changing. The patient must try again; the practitioner must try again. When patients return to their old behaviour, apply the same principles to once again engender change: raise the subject, explore importance and raise confidence, and discuss action options.

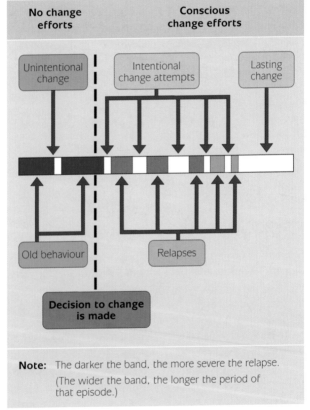

Note: The darker the band, the more severe the relapse.
(The wider the band, the longer the period of that episode.)

Figure 3. Natural history of relapses.

How do you know when the relapses are really over?

Many clinicians and researchers consider 6 months without relapse to be a point beyond which a new healthy behaviour is considered to be permanent, or in "maintenance".[44] But this is arbitrary. This time period varies from person to person and from behaviour to behaviour. One smoker might never relapse after first quitting; others might need eight or 10 attempts before maintaining change. We believe the most reasonable stance to take about relapse is to keep the following points in mind:

- Relapse is not inevitable when people seek permanent change, but it is the rule rather than the exception.
- Relapses should not be considered catastrophic. Don't convey despair.
- Relapses can teach patients what works and what does not, which is important knowledge for achieving lasting change.
- Mindlessly trying again without improving your plan is unproductive.
- To stop relapsing, people must figure out how to meet their essential needs without resorting to the old behaviour. Was it stress reduction? Fun? Companionship? Spiritual needs? Emotional needs? Others?
- After a relapse, reapply the same change principles found in this book.
- The mechanics of relapses are such that they begin long before the unwanted behaviour returns (see lightning metaphor below).
- The longer one maintains a new behaviour without relapse, the lower are one's chances of relapsing.
- Practitioners should repeatedly ask about and praise change rather than taking it for granted.

Metaphors to raise patients' confidence after relapses

Metaphors are helpful for consoling patients who have relapsed and encouraging them to try again. A good metaphor illustrates the mechanics of relapses, normalizes set backs, and renews hope. After reading these, try creating a few of your own.

Relapses are not like lightning striking

No. Relapses seldom happen by accident; but it seems this way to patients. This seemingly random, unpredictable nature of relapses—like lightning striking–can be very discouraging. To reassure patients, tell them that relapses actually begin well before the problem behaviour returns. Consider the patient with diabetes who successfully eliminates high fat foods for 4 months but then eventually relapses to his baseline high fat diet. In reviewing the relapse with him, you might both discover that he unwittingly dismantled his new habit in gradual steps. First, he returned to his favourite high fat restaurant, where it was difficult to order low fat food. Next, the discipline of pre-emptively buying low fat, tasty substitute foods for snacking at home dropped off—too inconvenient to go out of his way to that special store. So he began snacking again from high fat convenience stores. Before he realized it, he was back to his old ways. This raises hope that future relapses are preventable, not mysterious.

Changing old habits is like putting out a forest fire

Stopping an old, unwanted lifestyle behaviour is less like throwing a toggle switch and more like putting out a forest fire. After the flames are extinguished, a few embers may glow underground. Sometimes they ignite new brushfires. But these are easier to put out, as long as the patient acts again before his momentum is lost. The message is, small fires are normal, but keep stomping them out.

Relapses are like springtime rains

With informed and consistent effort, relapses gradually subside in frequency and intensity just as rainy winter days are replaced by sunny summer ones. Relapses can be seen as springtime rains, unwanted but likely to subside if one keeps trying and is patient.

A checklist to use before returning to action

When patients are ready to try again, practitioners can help by reviewing with their patients the following checklist. This is simply a menu of ideas for patients to choose from. It gives them a chance to select an idea or strategy that gives them the confidence to try again.

- *How will you meet your essential needs this time?*
- *What worked well the last time that you will repeat this time?*
- *One thing I will **stop doing** the next time I try (learned from previous effort).*
- *One thing I will **start doing** the next time I try (learned from previous effort).*
- *Did you link any of your new behaviours to automatic habits you already had? If not, how will you do this next time?*

Medication adherence

"To write prescriptions is easy, but to come to an understanding with people is hard".

Franz Kafka in *A Country Doctor*.

The prevalence of non-adherence

It is estimated that 50% of patients with chronic conditions do not take their medicines as prescribed — or indeed at all.[45] At the individual patient level, medication adherence is an integral feature of lifestyle and behaviour change, for two reasons. First, taking medications as prescribed is, in and of itself, one of

---

Evidence of the prevalence of non-adherence

Antihypertensives: A review of 14 studies of over 10,000 hypertensive patients found that 50% dropped out of treatment and only two thirds of those remaining took enough medication to control their blood pressure.[46]

Immuno-suppressive agents: After receiving organ transplants, 18% of renal transplant patients did not take their immuno-suppressive medication as prescribed. 91% of these patients suffered organ rejection or death compared to 18% of those adhering to the medication regimen.[47]

Cardiac agents: Among 2175 patients who had sustained a myocardial infarction, those not complying well with their medicine regimen were 2.5 times more likely to die within a year as those complying well.[48]

Metered dose inhalers: Poor adherence to asthma medication regimens has been repeatedly demonstrated by the medical literature to range from 30–70% in patients of all ages.[49]

Tuberculosis medication: Non-compliance with anti-tuberculosis treatment was 69% in a symptomatic HIV cohort.[46]

Multiple diseases: Electronic motoring of medication devices has identified compliance rates of under 50% for heart disease, asthma, epilepsy, diabetes mellitus, ankylosing spondylitis, depression and schizophrenia.[46]

Box 28. Medication non-adherence.

several lifestyle changes that patients with chronic illness must face. Second, taking certain medications as prescribed can greatly improve one's chances of successfully making other lifestyle changes involving healthier habits.

This thinking is high on the government agenda in the UK, where serious and promising medication adherence initiatives are underway. The Audit Commission report on Medicines Management[45] has established the expectation that by 2004 every primary care trust (PCT) is expected to have developed a Medication Management Strategy. The medication management pilot schemes currently under way in the UK and the overall progress PCTs are making in this direction is indeed encouraging. The Working Party of The Royal Pharmaceutical Society of Great Britain has clearly stated that a central part of

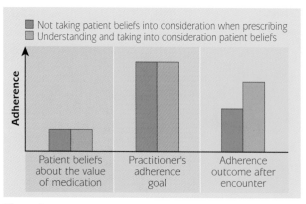

Figure 4. Maximizing adherence by understanding patient beliefs about medication.

successful medicines management is the shared partnership between doctor and patient.[50] This chapter focuses on this partnership.

Medication non-adherence has been defined in many ways. Here are a few examples: not filling the prescription, filling it but never taking it, and taking it inconsistently, incompletely, at the wrong times, or with the wrong foods.[51]

A reasonable goal: Maximal, not perfect, adherence

This section discusses and offers tips about one factor that can influence adherence: *patient beliefs*. For a more comprehensive approach to medication adherence, see *Rapid Reference to Compliance*.[51]

As with other behaviour changes, adherence varies along a continuum; it's not an all-or-nothing phenomenon. There may always be a gap between the degree of adherence practitioners hope for and what they actually get. A reasonable goal is to reduce this gap. The value of understanding patient beliefs and taking them into consideration when prescribing is illustrated in the Figure 4. This idea is supported by the research cited in the rest of this section.

Main ideas about adherence

Using people skills versus medical knowledge: in a study of patient satisfaction and medication adherence, the effects of practitioners' interpersonal skill levels were compared to the number of teaching statements they made during an encounter. Practitioner's interpersonal skills included conveying respect and understanding for the patient's views about medication. For patients with chronic illness, there was a strong association between interpersonal skills and patient recall of medication information, given the same number of teaching statements made. Medication adherence was increased by increased patient

The effects of patient beliefs on adherence

Antihypertensives: Adherence to antihypertension medication was compared among two groups of women: those who believed in the existence of the biomedical disease of hypertension and those whose concept of hypertension had a folk aetiology and disagreed with medical wisdom. Only 27% of patients who shared their doctor's concept of hypertension were non-adherent, compared to 63% of those who believed in the folk illness view.[52]

Box 29. Patients beliefs on adherence.

What are the common patient beliefs affecting importance and confidence?

- I shouldn't take this medicine because my body will become immune to its effects. Then, nothing will work. So I won't take it unless I get sicker .

- This drug is "unnatural". Unnatural agents are more harmful to me than "natural" medicines, such as herbal remedies.

- I will become addicted to this medicine.

- The costs of taking this medicine (e.g. financial, side effects, inconvenience) outweigh the benefits (e.g. uncertain survival).

- I don't need my antidepressant every day, only when I'm feeling down.

- I'm just not as susceptible to diabetes as others are. After all, it affects everyone differently.

- If I take this medicine, my body won't learn to combat my medical condition on its own.

- I need to discontinue this medication to test if it was really working

(All of the above from Working Party of The Royal Pharmaceutical Society of Great Britain[50].)

- It will make me a weak person to have to depend on a pill to solve my problems.[53]

- All pharmaceuticals are harmful, not only drugs of abuse such as cocaine or heroin.[54]

- The cons of taking this drug far outweigh the pros.[55]

- This disease isn't as serious as my doctor thinks.[56]

Box 30. Common patient beliefs.

satisfaction and recall of medication information.[37] Although the exact mechanism is not known, it seems that conveying an understanding of the patient can enhance adherence.

Once is not enough: Among studies of interventions that succeeded in improving medication adherence, a consistent finding is that improvements decay over time if not repeated regularly.[57-60] At every visit, when reviewing medications with patients, be sure to reassess adherence. Praise adherence and intervene with non-adherence.

The world of theory and evidence

The type of behaviour change counselling we have advocated in this book is linked to empirically supported theories of behaviour change. Below are thumbnail sketches of each theory and part of the evidence supporting them. The references provided will guide you to in-depth readings.

Summaries of major behaviour change theories and their supporting evidence

Humanistic theory states that people are powerfully motivated to seek health and happiness and will automatically do so, unless they are blocked through relationships with others who provide them with only conditional acceptance and regard. Three conditions in helping relationships are necessary for change to occur: warmth, accurate understanding of the person by the helper, and unconditional positive regard.[61–63]

Example: A patient-centred interviewing style was found to: increase patient satisfaction, increase medication adherence, reduce blood pressure, improve postoperative recovery and improve blood sugar management among diabetics.[64–66]

Transtheoretical model of change

Also called the Stage of Change model (SOM), states that readiness to change varies along a continuum consisting of five stages: precontemplation, contemplation, preparation, action, and maintenance.[44,67] For people at each of these stages, the motivational tasks for preparing for the next stage differ greatly. One value of the model is it reminds clinicians to match their interventions to their patients' readiness levels. Each person varies in her readiness to change each of many different health behaviours and for different goals regarding only one behaviour.

Example: Although many obese patients are ready to plan for losing weight, they vary widely in how ready each patient is to change each of these behaviours: caloric intake, vegetable and fruit intake, and planned exercise. So providers and patients must be clear about which target behaviour they are discussing.[10]

Readiness to change and importance and confidence

The SOM model is a powerful descriptive tool for understanding the process of change and reminding practitioners to accept that many people aren't ready to take action. However, there is not yet enough empirical evidence to dictate which counselling techniques to use for each stage. We are keen not to complicate a simplified guide to behaviour change counselling by weaving into it the SOM Model. For this book, we consider importance and confidence to be two main components of motivation or readiness, so we focus on them. As stated previously, as importance and confidence increase, readiness is thought to increase.

Example: Smokers frequently tell us that they don't really consider themselves ready to quit smoking, even though it is very important to them, because they are not confident of their ability to succeed.

Self-efficacy theory and social cognitive theory

These state that in addition to learning by practising a behaviour, people learn vicariously by observing others. People are most likely to copy behaviour they see in others if they identify with them and like them. People have control over their behaviours largely due to how they think about them. Self-efficacy is a state in which one thinks one has the ability to perform a behaviour successfully. Self-efficacy in the same person varies across different situations. People need to believe in their skills to succeed, and short-term success can raise this belief.[68–69]

The fine line between self-efficacy and overconfidence

Self-efficacy is confidence that one can achieve one's objectives. We should maximize self-efficacy before encouraging patients to attempt to change. But, there is a limit to how confident one can be without yet having experienced success. Self-efficacy is partly earned, based on a record of success and competency.[70] Overconfidence is an overestimation of one's ability to succeed in reaching unrealistic goals. It is at the heart of action–relapse cycle. It provokes poorly planned action and sets up people for disappointment after change has begun but unrealistic expectations have not been met. Common unrealistic expectations are beliefs that change will come more quickly, more easily, in greater magnitude, and will improve other areas of life more than is realistic.[71] Without sabotaging self-efficacy, practitioners must remain vigilant for overconfidence and help patients to set more realistic goals and expectations about changes they are about to undertake. When patients lower their expectations and demand less of themselves, their self-efficacy will increase because they sense their goals are reachable.[71]

Example: An obese patient begins another diet with fierce determination. She has the unrealistic expectations of easily and rapidly losing 50 pounds, hoping that she will then find a romantic partner. The weight drops at first but it soon levels out, leaving her discouraged and irritable much of the time. She begins to backslide and within 6 months weighs 7 pounds more than when she started. She needs help to lower her expectations (less weight lost more slowly, using a very careful plan to find ways to eat satisfying foods every day).

Self-determination theory

States that only autonomous or internal motivation results in long-term healthy behaviour change. Autonomous motivation means using one's own volition and self-initiation, and personally believing that behaviour change will cause improved health. External motivation comes from forces outside of people that pressure them to change, such as a health practitioner, employer, or family member.

Examples: Obese patients higher in internal motivation are more likely to lose weight.[75] Highly internally versus externally motivated diabetic patients are more likely to maintain glucose control.[76] And patients higher in internal motivation are more likely to stop smoking continuously for over 30 months when advised to quit by physicians.[77]

Other evidence supporting these theories

Advice isn't always called for: In American and British studies, smokers not ready to quit had, before seeing the doctor, made their own self-evaluations of the negative side of smoking and anticipated being advised by their doctors to do so. This advice caused patients to respond by shrugging it off, feeling guilty or feeling annoyed. Patients accepted counselling that conveyed a respectful tone; avoided preaching, and provided a caring, individualized approach.[72,73].

Merely giving patients education isn't enough: A review of 72 randomised trials over 20 years of self-management training interventions with type 2 diabetics concluded that knowledge alone is not enough to secure long-term behavioural change. Although a minimum threshold of patient knowledge about diabetes is needed, changes in attitude and motivation are more effective than knowledge in achieving metabolic control.[74]

Box 34. Additional evidence.

Outcome research

Part of the large body of behaviour change outcome research on brief interventions in medical settings is shown on pages 20–21. Theses studies addressed drinking, smoking, physical activity, and dietary change. We believe this promising evidence that modest behaviour change can be achieved with interventions lasting a relatively short period of time. However, few if any of these studies tested Behaviour Change Counselling as described on this book. The difference is that BCC emphasizes using counselling skills to elicit from the patient the argument in favour of change. BCC places greater emphasis on exploring the *why* of change than most other brief intervention methods.

Much closer to BCC in style and method is Motivational Interviewing. Two independent, systematic reviews have been conducted of a large number of randomized, controlled studies of adaptations of Motivational Interviewing for substance abuse, smoking, HIV, risk reduction, and diet and exercise.[78, 79] There was substantial evidence that MI is an effective substance abuse intervention method when used by clinicians who are non-specialists in substance abuse treatment. A smaller number of studies in the other three domains were mixed but promising.

References

1. Miller WR, Rollnick S. Motivational Interviewing: Preparing People for Change. New York: Guilford, 2002.

2. Rollnick S, Mason P, Butler C. Health Behaviour Change: A Guide for Practitioners. London: Churchill Livingstone, 1999.

3. Rollnick S, Allison J, Ballasiotes S *et al*. Variations on a theme: Motivational interviewing and its adaptations. In: Miller WR and Rollnick S, *Motivational Interviewing: Preparing People for change*. New York: Guilford, 2002.

4. McGinnis MJ, Foege WH. Actual causes of death in the United States. *JAMA* 1993; **270**: 2207–2212.

5. Office for National Statistics, UK. Statistics on smoking: England, (1998). http://www.doh.gov.uk/public/sb0017.htm

6. Thom TJ, Kannel WB, Silbershatz H, *et al*. Incidence, prevalence, and mortality of cardiovascular disease in the United States. In: RW Alexander, RD Schlant, V Fuster, editors. *Hurst's The Heart, Arteries and Veins*, 9th Edition. New York: McGraw-Hill, pp.3–16.

7. US Department of Health and Human Services. The health benefits of smoking cessation: A report of the Surgeon General. Atlanta GA: US Department of Health and Human Services 1990. DHHS Publication No. (CDC) 90–8416.

8. Stampfer MJ, Hu FB, Manson JE *et al*. Primary prevention of coronary heart disease in women through diet and lifestyle. *New Eng. J Med* 2000; **343**:16–22.

9. National Diabetes Data Group. *Diabetes in America*, 2nd Edition. Bethesda MD: National Institutes of Health, 1995.

10. Logue E, Suttjon K, Jarjoura D *et al*. Obesity management in primary care: assessment of readiness to change among 284 family practice patients. *J Am Bd of Fam Prac* 2000; **13**: 164–171.

11. Kujela UM, Kaprio J, Sarna S. Relationship of leisure-time physical activity and mortality. *JAMA* 1998; **275**: 440.

12. Saaddine JB, Engelgau MM, Beckles GL *et al*. A diabetes report card for the United States: quality of care in the 1990s. *An Int Med* 2002; **136**(8): 565–574.

13. Harris MI, Eastman RC, Cowie CC *et al.* Racial and ethnic differences in glycemic control of adults with type 2 diabetes. *Diabetes Care* **22**: 403–408.

14. American Diabetes Association Standards of medical care for patients with diabetes mellitus. *Diabetes Care* 1994; **17**(6): 616–623.

15. Arnsten JH, Demas PA, Grant RW *et al.* Impact of active drug use on antiretroviral therapy adherence and viral suppression in HIV-infected drug users. *J Gen Intern Med* 2002; **17**: 377–381.

16. Office for National Statistics, UK. Statistics on alcohol: England,1998. http://www.doh.gov.uk/public/sb0113.htm

17. Office for National Statistics, UK. Sun exposure:Adults behaviour and knowledge. ONS Omnibus Survey. http://www.doh.gov.uk/public/sun.htm

18. Stratton IM, Adler AI, Neil HA *et al.* Association of glycaemia with macrovascular and microvascular complications of type 2 diabetes (UKPDS 35): prospective observational study. *Br Med J* 2002; **321**(7258): 405–412.

19. Boule NG, Haddad E, Kenny GP *et al.* Effects of exercise on glycemic control and body mass in type 2 diabetes mellitus: a meta-analysis of controlled clinical trials. *JAMA* 2001; 286(10):1218–1227.

20. Diabetes Prevention Program Research Group. Reduction in the incidence of type 2 diabetes with lifestyle intervention or metformin. *New Eng J Med* 2002; **346**(6):393–403.

21. Kraemer KL, Maisto SA, Conigliaro J *et al.* Decreased alcohol consumption in outpatient drinkers is associated with improved quality of life and fewer alcohol-related consequences. *J Gen Intern Med* 2002; 17: 382–386.

22. Sacks FM, Svetkey LP, Vollmer WM *et al.* Effects on blood pressure of reduced dietary sodium and the Dietary Approaches to Stop Hypertension (DASH) diet. DASH-Sodium Collaborative Research Group. *New Engl J Med* 2001; **344**(1): 3–10.

23. Adams A, Ockene JK, Wheeler EV *et al* . Alcohol counselling: Physicians will do it. *J Gen Intern Med* 1998; **13**: 692–698.

24. Sobell LC, Sobell MB, Toneatto T *et al.* What triggers the resolution of alcohol problems without treatment. *Alcohol Clin Exp Res* 1993; **17**(2): 217–24.

25. Anderson P, Scott E. The effect of general practitioners' advice to heavy drinking men. *Br J Addict* 1992; **87**: 891–900.

26. Wallace P, Cutler S, Haines A. Randomised controlled trial of general practitioner intervention in patients with excessive alcohol consumption. BMJ 1998; **297**: 663–668.

27. Babor TF, Grant M. Project on Identification and management of alcohol-related problems. Report on Phase II: a randomized clinical trial of brief interventions in primary health care. Geneva: World Health Organization, 1992.

28. Nilssen O. The Tromso study: identification of and a controlled intervention on a population of early stage problem drinkers in primary health care. *Br J Addict* 1991; **84**: 1319–1327.

29. Maheswaran R, Beevers M, Gareth D. Effectiveness of advice to reduce alcohol consumption in hypertensive patients. *Hypertension* 1992; **19**: 79–84.

30. Kahan M, Wilson L, Becker L. Effectiveness of physician-based interventions with problem drinkers: A review. *Can Med Assoc J* 1995; **152**(6): 851-859.

31. Bien TH, Miller WR, Tonigan JM. Brief interventions for alcohol problems: A review, *Addiction* 1993; **88**: 315–316.

32. Law M , Tang JL . An analysis of the effectiveness of interventions intended to help people stop smoking. *Arch Intern Med* 1995; **155**(18): 1933–41.

33. Writing Group for the Activity Counseling Trial Research Group. Effects of physical activity counseling in primary care: the Activity Counseling Trial: a randomized controlled trial. *JAMA* 2001; **286**(6): 677–687.

34. Brunner E, White I, Thorogood M *et al*. Can dietary interventions change diet and cardiovascular risk factors? A meta-analysis of randomized controlled trials. *Am J Public Health* 1997; **87**(9):1415–1422.

35. Brehm SS, Brehm JW. Psychological reactance: A Theory of Freedom and Control. New York: Academic Press, 1981.

36. Prochaska J, DiClemente CC. Toward a comprehensive model of change. In: Miller WR, Heather N, editors. Treating Addictive Behaviors: Processes of Change. New York: Plenum, 1986, pp.3–27.

37. Bartlett EE, Grayson M, Barker R *et al*. The effects of physician communications skills on patient satisfaction, recall, and adherence. *J Chronic Disease* 1984; **37**(9): 755–764.

38. Stott NCH, Rollnick R, Rees MR, Pill RM. Innovation in clinical method: diabetes care and negotiating skills. *Fam Prac* 1995; **12**(4): 413–418.

39. Gollwitzer PM. Implementation intentions: Strong effects of simple plans. *Amer Psychol* 1999; **54**(7): 493–503.

40. Sheeran P, Orbell S. Implementation intentions and repeated behaviors: Augmenting the predictive validity of the theory of planned behaviour. *Eur J Soc Psychol* 1999; **29**: 349–370.

41. Sheeran P, Orbell S. Using implementation intentions to increase attendance for cervical cancer screening. Health Psychol 2000; **19**(3): 283–9.

42. Polansky, W. Diabetes burnout: What to do when you Can't Take it Anymore. Canada: American Diabetes Association, 1999.

43. Fletcher AM. *Sober for Good*. New York, Houghton Mifflin, 2001.

44. Prochaska J, DiClemente CC. Stages and processes of self-change of smoking: towards an integrated model of change. *J Consul Clin Psychol* 1983; **51**: 390–395.

45. Audit Commission Report: *A Spoonful of Sugar—Medicines Management in NHS Hospitals*. Audit Commission, 2001.

46. Dunbar-Jacob J, Dwyer K, Dunning EJ. Compliance with anti-hypertensive regimen: A review of the research in the 1980s. *Ann Behav Med* 1991; **13**(1): 31–39.

47. Rjovelli M, Palmeri D, Vossler E *et al*. Non-compliance in organ transplant recipients. *Transplant Proc* 1989; **21**(1): 833–834.

48. Horwitz RI, Viscoli CM, Berkman L *et al*. Treatment adherence and risk of death after a myocardial infarction. *Lancet* 1990; **336**: 542–545.

49. Rand CS, Wise RA . Measuring adherence to asthma medication regimens. *Am J Respir Crit Care Med* 1994; **149**: S69–S76.

50. Working Party of The Royal Pharmaceutical Society of Great Britain. *From compliance to concordance: Achieving shared goals*

77. Williams GC, Gagne M, Ryan RM *et al*. Facilitating autonomous motivation for smoking cessation. *Health Psych* 2001; **21**: 40–50.

78. Dunn CW, DeRoo L, Rivara FP. The use of brief interventions adapted from motivational interviewing across behavioural domains: A systematic review. *Addiction* 2001; **96**: 1725–1742.

79. Burke BL, Arkowitz H, Dunn CW. The efficacy of motivational interviewing and its adaptations. In: WR Miller, S Rollnick, editors *Motivational Interviewing: Preparing People for Change*. New York: Guilford, 2002, pp. 270–283.

Further reading

Ashenden R, Silagy C, Weller D. A systematic review of the effectiveness of promoting lifestyle change in general practice. *Fam Pract* 1997; **14**(2): 160–176.

Bayer Institute for Health Care Communication. Managing medication: *Improving health by creating partnerships. A workshop syllabus for pharmacists*. West Haven, CT, 1999.

Handmaker NS, Miller WR, Manicke M. Findings of a pilot study of motivational interviewing with pregnant drinker. *J Studies Alcohol* 1999; **60**: 285–287.

Miller WR, Benefield RG, Tonigan J. Enhancing motivation for change in problem drinking: A controlled comparison of two therapist styles, *J Consult Clin Psychol* 1993; **61**(3), 455–461.

Rollnick S. Behaviour change in practice: Targeting individuals. *Intern J of Obesity Related Metabolic* 1996; **20**(suppl): S22–S26.

Rollnick S, Kinnersley P, Stott N. Methods of helping patients with behaviour change. *Br Med J* 1993; **307**(6897): 188–90.

Ways, P. *Take Charge of your Health: The Guide to Personal Health Competence*. Vermont: Stephen Greene Press Inc, distributed by Viking Penguin, 1985.

Helpful internet resources

Medicines Partnership. Training for health professionals, demonstration partnership projects, reviews of published research on compliance and concordance, patient views and patient-targeted information: www.medicines-partnership.org

The Motivational Interviewing Page. A repository of resources on motivational interviewing, including links, training resources, reprints and videotapes: www.motivationalinterview.org

The Bayer Institute For Health Care Communication. The Institute works with health care organizations to conduct research and provide educational opportunities to make it possible for clinicians to develop the communication skills they need to be effective: www.bayerinstitute.com

The Centre for Motivation & Change: A non-profit foundation providing training, consulting and education in the fields of chronic disease management, addictions, lifestyle change and health promotion, compliance with medication, stress-management and organisational change: www.tomaatnet.nl/%7Erikbes/cmc.htm

A behaviour change counselling training videotape based on *Health Behaviour Change* (book by Rollnick, Mason, Butler, 1999) is available from: www.jeffallison.co.uk/index.htm

Appendix

Bupropion: Nicotine replacement therapy for smoking cessation. Provides a regulated taper from nicotine and reduces nicotine cravings during early abstinence.

Disulfiram: Assists drinkers to abstain from alcohol by causing nausea, vomiting, headaches, flushing, and palpitations if any alcohol is consumed.

Campral: Reduces intensity of alcohol cravings and frequency of drinking. Available in Europe, but not in the US.

Naltrexone: Helps drinkers to abstain by reducing subjective cravings for alcohol and lessening the intensity of relapses if they occur.

Naltrexone: An opioid antagonist that facilitates abstinence by blocking the euphoric effects of heroin or other opiates.

Phentermine: Reduces appetite by stimulating CNS activity.

Orlistat: Helps with weight loss by slowing fat absorption.

Sibutramine and diethylpropion: Reduce appetite by lowering norepenephrine, serotonin, and dopamine reuptake.

Other antidepressants: Can assist lifestyle behaviour change by reducing depression, which can lead to discouragement, low activation levels, and difficulty concentrating on complex tasks.

Index

Since the major subject of this book is behaviour change, entries have been kept to a minimum under this term: readers are advised to seek more specific entries.

This index is in letter-by-letter order, whereby spaces and hyphens in main entries are excluded from the alphabetization process. Page numbers followed by 'f' indicate figures: page numbers followed by 'b' indicate boxes.